Hospital-related malnutrition

Susan Holmes

PhD, BSc, SRN, FRSH, CMS

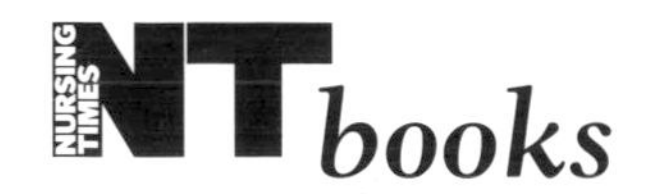

Emap Healthcare Ltd
Greater London House
Hampstead Road
London NW1 7EJ

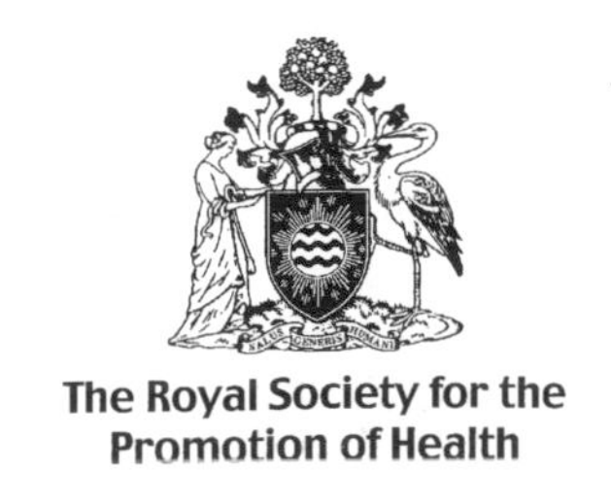

The Royal Society for the Promotion of Health

Nursing Times Clinical Monographs are authoritative, concise, single subject publications designed to provide a critical review of material that will be of value to practising nurses, midwives and health visitors. Their authors, all experts in their field, are asked to be challenging and thought-provoking and to stimulate reflection on current practice. *Nursing Times* Clinical Monographs do not seek to be exhaustive reviews but up-to-date overviews; their critical and evaluative nature is designed to promote best practice through consideration of current evidence.

Topics for publication are decided by the editorial advisory board, with input from practitioners. Monographs are then commissioned as near as possible to the publication date to ensure that the information they contain is the latest available. All manuscripts are reviewed by a board member and a clinician working in the field covered.

Every three months, 12-15 new monographs will be published. They will cover subjects suggested by practitioners (see bottom of page) and any major new developments in the field of nursing care. Each publication will be on sale for a limited time, after which it will be withdrawn and, if necessary, replaced with an updated version.

Suggestions for future titles are welcome and should be sent to Simon Seljeflot at NT Books, Emap Healthcare, Greater London House, London NW1 7EJ

Nursing Times Clinical Monographs do not seek to be an exhaustive review of the topic but provide an overview of current evidence, stimulating discussion and debate.

Hospital-related malnutrition

Susan Holmes, PhD, BSc, SRN, FRSH, CMS

Good nutrition is central to optimum health and to the recovery from illness, yet repeated reports have revealed the many difficulties associated with feeding hospital patients, and clinical surveys continue to reveal an unacceptably high incidence of malnutrition among sick people. Although the evolution of malnutrition during illness is complex and frequently reflects the severity of the patients' disease or the damaging effects of the therapies applied to them, this is not always the case, and many other factors may contribute to its development. These are explored below. The provision of food and drink to patients is complex. While nurses are at the 'sharp end' of patient feeding and clearly carry responsibility for ensuring that patients are eating adequately, the provision of food to patients involves most hospital departments and all health care professionals. Food is an important part of the 'hotel' services received by hospital patients and a central component of their overall satisfaction with hospital care. This means that food, food service and nutrition itself are important determinants of clinical outcome, cost-effectiveness of hospital care and patient satisfaction with the quality of care received

Butterworth, writing in *Nutrition Today* in 1974, revealed a significant incidence of malnutrition in a wide variety of hospital patients in the USA, dubbing this the 'skeleton in the hospital closet'. He also demonstrated the way in which hospitals themselves contributed to the development of the problem. This controversial publication raised many eyebrows among practising clinicians on both sides of the Atlantic who found it difficult to believe that malnutrition was a significant problem in clinical environments.

The 1970s saw a plethora of work on medical and surgical patients, in both the USA and the UK, concluding that malnutrition affects up to 50% (or more) of patients hospitalised for two weeks or longer (Bistrian et al, 1974; 1976; Hill et al, 1977; McWhirter and Pennington, 1994), thus confirming Butterworth's findings. These and many other studies have shown that patients with evidence of malnutrition have significantly longer hospital stays and higher rates of both morbidity and mortality (Reilly et al, 1987; Anderson et al, 1985), thus consuming more hospital resources and, of course, increasing the costs of hospital care (McCamish, 1993); this may be reversed by treatment (Bastow et al, 1983; Rana et al, 1992; Tucker, 1996).

Still further work revealed that patients with low levels of circulating proteins experienced greater levels of both surgical (Windsor and Hill, 1988) and medical (Potter et al, 1995) complications. Indeed, McCamish (1993) suggested that patients with malnutrition were two to three times more likely to develop complications than those who were adequately nourished.

Yet, even in 1994, the work of McWhirter and Pennington drew further attention to the problem of hospital-related malnutrition, followed by the Association of Community Health Councils' report *Hungry in Hospitals* (1997), which showed that many patients were receiving insufficient food to assuage their hunger. Similarly, the Patients' Association (1993) has highlighted the problems of unappealing institutional meals, while Mennell et al (1994) discussed the lack of attention to the social context and organisation of food provision. It is, perhaps, not surprising that the

Notes

Relatives' Association receives continual complaints about the quality of hospital food and the failure to feed those requiring help.

The question is why this continues in the 1990s when both health care and nutritional knowledge are so advanced and continual developments in food science and technology have significantly increased the availability of a wide variety of high-quality and nutritious foods. There is also a wealth of information about consumer preferences and patient satisfaction that should, when taken together, make it possible to provide foods that meet individual preferences as well as nutritional requirements.

The problem is that the majority of work regarding the quality of hospital food is based on studies that address matters of personal taste or satisfaction, rather than nutritional adequacy (Allison, 1996). Similarly, although significant sums of money are spent on hospital food, Allison (1996) suggested that the nutritional care of the majority of patients has suffered from the separation of budgets into 'hotel' and 'treatment' costs, with the effect that the supply of food in hospitals is viewed as a 'supplement' to clinical care rather than as an integral part of it unless a therapeutic diet is required.

Thus, although hospital catering guidelines (NHS Executive, 1996) were designed to ensure continuous improvements in food service, the matter of patient feeding requires a great deal of consideration. The importance of nutrition, and the deleterious effects of malnutrition, have long been recognised, yet the condition persists; that it still exists makes Butterworth's 'skeleton' well worth revisiting.

Defining malnutrition

The word malnutrition literally means bad nutrition and so can be applied to any condition in which there is a nutritional disorder. It may, therefore, reflect undernutrition, due to an inadequate food intake, or overnutrition, due to excessive food consumption. It may also be used to refer to deficiencies of specific nutrients (for example, vitamins or minerals) or a dietary imbalance due to a disproportionate intake of particular foods or food components (Keller, 1993).

Although Keller's work focused on the problems of undernutrition, those associated with overnutrition (overweight or obesity) must not be overlooked, since this condition may mask specific nutritional deficiencies. Indeed, nutritional deficits may be present in the overweight patient even in the absence of overall loss of body weight.

Thus, the term malnutrition, as used here, refers to the wasting condition resulting from a deficiency of protein and calories (energy) accompanied by varying degrees of trace nutrient (vitamin and mineral) deficiencies. Such protein-energy malnutrition (PEM) is the most common form of malnutrition seen in hospital patients (American Society of Parenteral and Enteral Nutrition, 1993).

Types of malnutrition

There are two main types of PEM — severe calorie deficiency (marasmus) and maladaptive states combining protein deficiency with metabolic stress (kwashiorkor). At times these conditions can be combined, resulting in marasmic kwashiorkor.

As can be seen from Table 1 opposite, marasmus is a chronic disorder rather than an acute condition and represents a prolonged period of calorie deprivation that results in cachexia. Illnesses producing such malnutrition are, therefore, primarily chronic conditions, such as cancer, chronic respiratory disorders or cardiac disease. The diagnosis is confirmed by the clinical evidence of significant depletion of body fat and muscle combined with a prolonged period of caloric deprivation. This is manifested clinically by markedly reduced skinfold thickness, which reflects the loss of subcutaneous fat (energy reserves), and reduced arm muscle circumference, with associated muscle-wasting, reflecting the loss of protein from skeletal muscles. Such

Table 1. Types of malnutrition

Type	Contributory factors	Time to develop	Clinical features	Clinical course	Mortality
Marasmus	Reduced calorie intake	Months to years	Starved appearance; weight less than 80% of ideal body weight; triceps skinfold thickness less than 5mm; midarm muscle circumference less than 15cm	Response to stress is reasonably preserved	Mortality low unless related to the underlying disease
Kwashiorkor	Reduced protein intake associated with stress	Weeks	Apparently well-nourished; hair plucks easily; oedema	Prone to infection; wound healing is poor; pressure sores and skin breakdown are likely	Mortality rate is high

wasting also affects internal organs, such as the heart, kidneys and liver.

Kwashiorkor in hospital patients is, in contrast, primarily associated with acute and life-threatening conditions, such as significant trauma and sepsis, which are associated with a hypermetabolic (catabolic) state that increases demand for both protein and energy at a time when dietary intake is often reduced. In such circumstance, kwashiorkor can develop rapidly.

The combined form of PEM (marasmic kwashiorkor) may develop when physiological stress is superimposed on chronically starved individuals.

Trace nutrient deficiency

Although deficiencies of vitamins and minerals may affect any malnourished patient, such deficits may also arise in patients experiencing acute or chronic illness. Such individuals often develop abnormalities of micronutrients through, for example, diarrhoea, drainage, exudate or other external secretions. Others may have increased requirements for particular nutrients, such as a heightened demand for vitamins during periods of sepsis. Such deficiencies particularly affect nutrients that are stored in the body in only limited amounts (for example, the water-soluble vitamins — the vitamin B complex and vitamin C).

Why is malnutrition unrecognised?

Malnutrition, when it occurs in the UK, is most often the result of an underlying disease process. Its continuing development often results from a failure to identify its presence or to recognise and/or meet the increased nutritional needs of sick patients (British Dietetic Association, 1996; Rademaker et al, 1996). It has been suggested that the failure to recognise the potential for malnutrition, either on admission or during the hospital stay, reflects the fact that neither nurses nor doctors are trained to anticipate it (Lennard-Jones, 1992).

For example, Parker et al (1992) showed that medical students know little about nutrition, while Philen et al (1992) revealed that doctors, like other members of the general public, are readily misled by the inaccurate advertising of nutritional products. Similarly, Mulliner et al (1995) showed that many midwives acknowledged their limitations with regard to the provision of nutritional information to the extent that they feel unable to fulfil their role of supporting pregnant women owing to an inadequate level of knowledge. Such facts must be of concern in modern day health care.

Since knowledgeable and motivated

Notes

Notes

staff are the key to the effective recognition, prevention and treatment of malnutrition, this lack of knowledge, or even simple unawareness, may have significant ramifications for patients (Taylor and Goodinson-McLaren, 1993; Department of Health, 1994; English National Board, 1995). Yet, as nutrition is given low priority in both nursing and medical education and training (Lennard-Jones, 1992; Department of Health, 1994), this is not surprising. Neither is it surprising that nutritional abnormalities, or even poor intake, are 'often not even considered in the hospital setting' (Reilly et al, 1996) and are believed to be 'so basic that they are taken for granted, sometimes even to the point of neglect' (Clark, 1980).

The importance of nutrition has, however, been recognised, and it is now recommended that a greater level of both theoretical and practical training should be included at both diploma and undergraduate level (Lennard-Jones, 1992; Department of Health, 1994; English National Board, 1995).

However, not all cases of malnutrition arise in hospital; a significant number of patients are malnourished on admission (Dickerson, 1986; McWhirter and Pennington, 1994). Malnutrition particularly affects those with chronic debilitating conditions affecting, for example, the gastrointestinal tract, which interfere with food ingestion or digestion and absorption (Dickerson, 1986) or those with neurological deficits resulting in dysphagia. Similarly, patients with cancer or other long-term disease may be at nutritional disadvantage. Older adults, particularly the recently bereaved (especially widowers), the socially isolated, those with mental or sensory impairment (Holmes, 1994) and the 'very old' (those over 80) (Department of Health, 1992) are especially vulnerable to nutritional depletion.

Although affected individuals may well have a low food intake, even consumption of apparently adequate amounts of food does not mean that they will not have micronutrient deficiencies (subclinical deficiencies) caused by dietary imbalance or vitamin losses resulting during food preparation and storage (Dickerson, 1986).

Deficiencies of vitamin B_1 (thiamine), vitamin C (ascorbic acid) and folic acid are common in older people (Schorah et al, 1974; Puxty, 1985) and may persist unless supplementation is given; hospital diets are known to be, at best, adequate only for maintenance and not repletion. Indeed, studies of older adults undergoing orthopaedic surgery have demonstrated that post-operative food consumption may provide less than 50% of the nutrients recommended for healthy people of the same age (Older and Dickerson, 1982; Dickerson et al, 1986).

Other surveys (for example, Simon, 1991) similarly revealed that the food served to patients may be deficient in one or more essential nutrients, including not only energy (calories) but also nutrients such as folic acid, iron and vitamin D.

The importance of such findings cannot be over-emphasised, since it cannot be assumed that a nutritionally adequate diet is always available to the hospital patient. Far from promoting recovery, the diet provided may promote pre-existing deficiencies exacerbated still further by surgery, which increases the requirement for both vitamin B_1 and vitamin C.

Aetiology of malnutrition

As has been shown, malnutrition in hospital patients is most commonly the effect of an underlying illness. It may develop due to the following factors:

- Decreased dietary intake;
- Increased nutrient requirements;
- Impaired ability to absorb, utilise or metabolise nutrients.

It may be exacerbated by a variety of psychosocial factors, by admission to hospital and/or by the treatment the patient receives.

Decreased dietary intake

Food consumption and, hence, nutrient intake may be inhibited by a wide variety of factors, including a range of physical symptoms (Table 2 above) and various psychosocial factors.

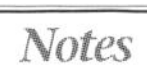

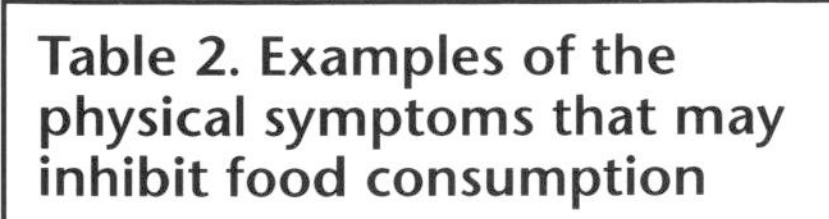

Table 2. Examples of the physical symptoms that may inhibit food consumption

- Anorexia
- Dysphagia
- Nausea and vomiting
- Taste changes
- Tooth decay and/or peridontal disease
- Oral mucositis (stomatitis)
- Diarrhoea/constipation
- Pain

For example, many patients develop dysphagia due to anatomical obstruction or neurological damage. Food intake is clearly reduced in those who experience nausea and/or vomiting, which may result from primary disease or from its treatment. Those with chronic ill health, such as many older people, often have an impaired appetite exacerbated by, for example, anxiety, depression or drug therapy. Impaired taste sensation may potentiate anorexia, particularly in the presence of malignancy (Holmes and Dickerson, 1987) or as a consequence of drug therapy.

Other possible causes of taste change include deficiencies of vitamin A, the vitamin B complex or the trace element zinc. Neurological disease and/or uraemia may also be contributory factors (Taylor and Goodinson-McLaren, 1993). Other factors that may restrict food consumption include gastrointestinal and respiratory disorders or malignant disease.

Clearly gastrointestinal conditions may affect food ingestion, digestion or absorption. For example, oral disorders, such as tooth decay and/or peridontal disease, may make eating both difficult and painful. Affected individuals often substitute soft, low-fibre foods for fresh fruit and vegetables or wholegrain cereals, thus distorting the dietary balance. Similarly, dysphagia and oesophageal disorders may result in distressing symptoms that may significantly reduce food consumption (Sonies et al, 1988), while symptoms such as nausea, vomiting and diarrhoea may both reduce intake and inhibit absorption. Constipation may cause abdominal pain and distension, thus reducing the appetite and, again, restricting nutrient availability.

Other examples include peptic ulceration and intestinal infection (or other inflammatory conditions), which may significantly affect both the patient's ability and willingness to eat as well as digestion and the absorption of nutrients. Hypochlorhydria will impair the digestion of protein and decrease absorption of both calcium and iron.

Respiratory diseases, such as chronic obstructive pulmonary disease (COPD) or pulmonary oedema, may cause severe dyspnoea, which often leads to an inability to eat without an associated increase in respiratory distress. Conversely, undernutrition may worsen respiratory difficulty (Arora and Rochester, 1962; Doekel et al, 1976), thus creating a vicious circle.

Hypermetabolism, often associated with COPD, may contribute to significant weight loss that may affect as many as 40% of patients with the condition (Wilson, 1990), while the production of significant amounts of sputum/mucus will decrease appetite and reduce the palatability of food.

Similarly, malignancy causes many symptoms that, when combined with the primary disease, exacerbate nutritional decline and result in significant morbidity and mortality. Both cancer and its treatment may contribute to the development of malnutrition, although in that case undernutrition reflects not only a reduced food consumption but also an increased demand for nutrients.

Many tumours are 'parasitic' and draw nutrients from the host. When food consumption fails to meet the nutritional needs of both the host and the tumour, body stores are catabolised. Moreover, malignancy itself induces profound metabolic changes that significantly affect the metabolism and utilisation of nutrients, resulting in a marked increase in the demand for energy and leading to depletion of body fat and protein that exacerbates weight loss and potentiates cachexia.

Notes

Hospitalisation

The preceding discussion provides examples of the way in which a patient's health status and his/her general condition may contribute to the aetiology of malnutrition. This may be intensified by the act of hospitalisation which may, in itself, adversely affect eating behaviour. For example, removal from the familiar environment of home, combined with the 'alien' surroundings of a hospital ward, may cause significant stress over and above that caused by illness *per se*. The surroundings and routines are far removed from patients' normal experiences, they may be anxious about what will happen and they become dependent on others for their care, their food provision and all other needs. All such factors may contribute to a reduced interest in food.

Evidence has shown that food consumption can be improved when patients are involved in planning their diet, have some control over food selection and feel responsible for following the advice they are given (Maras and Adolphi, 1985). Such involvement is, however, not always possible in the hospital setting.

For many patients, particularly older adults, meal times are the only event in the day to look forward to. Thus every attempt should be made to ensure that meal times are as pleasant as possible, a time that can be enjoyed and not a time that is simply regarded as another task that must be completed (Wainwright, 1978).

Institutional meals, however, are rarely pleasant social occasions and, as a captive population, patients have little control over food patterns, methods of preparation and times of eating, all of which often differ markedly from their normal food habits.

Patients are often left to eat in isolation; this may, in itself, restrict consumption. Eating in bed can be difficult; food intake may be limited by exasperation or frustration (Dickerson, 1986). Such factors, combined with the expectation of poor-quality hospital food (Association of Community Health Councils, 1997) may provoke food refusal. Alternatively, patients may refuse to eat particular foods or comply with dietary advice for religious or cultural reasons (Farb and Armelagos, 1980). Stress itself may be both a cause and a consequence of inadequate food consumption.

Unnecessarily prolonged starvation may be an additional factor in the development of undernutrition. For example, although investigations are essential they often result in patients missing their meals. Indeed, evidence has revealed that between 11% and 27% of all hospital meals are missed by patients (Eastwood, 1997) and that clinical investigations accounted for 7.6% of these. More than 92% of the total were, however, due to illness and/or the quality or taste of the food provided. This may be further exacerbated by visits by phlebotomists or medical personnel at meal times, since these are known to significantly reduce food consumption in some patients (Deutekom et al, 1991).

Although missing meals is sometimes unavoidable, it is essential that alternative arrangements are made to ensure that food intake is maintained at an appropriate level. This is often difficult to achieve and dietetic referral may be needed.

Hygiene regulations may prohibit both preparation and storage of food in ward kitchens (Garrow, 1994). This means that those patients who have to fast overnight and are absent from the ward at lunch may wait as long as 24 hours between meals. Postoperative patients may wait even longer without any form of nutritional support.

It is not surprising that many patients are vulnerable to at least some degree of nutritional depletion (Williams et al, 1989; Garrow, 1994; McWhirter and Pennington, 1994). This situation is exacerbated when appropriate help is not made available during meals or when nutritionally adequate alternatives are not offered to those refusing or unable to eat a meal for whatever reason. Nutritional status will, inevitably, decline.

Some patients may be physically handicapped and unable to manipulate cutlery. Food that is not cut up for them will not be eaten. Patient feeding may

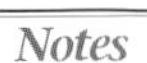

be delegated to unqualified staff who may lack the knowledge and/or skills necessary to help those with complex eating difficulties, and studies have found that food is, not uncommonly, placed outside the patient's reach and later removed untouched (Dickerson et al, 1986). When asked whether she had wanted the food one patient said: 'Yes, but I couldn't reach it'.

Interestingly, such factors may be exacerbated still further by the method of food service employed. For example, in a study exploring the meal-time care provided to patients in medical wards, Carr and Mitchell (1991) demonstrated that a meal-delivery system (plated meals) intended to 'free' nurses from serving patients' meals not only reduced patient choice, in terms of portion sizes, but also adversely affected nursing involvement in aspects of meal times, such as checking the patients' well-being, observing feeding problems and providing assistance.

Treatment-related effects

One of the factors both rarely considered and poorly understood by health care professionals is the interaction between drugs and nutrition. Some interactions are more significant than others and can result in adverse reactions to drugs, drug toxicity or the therapeutic failure of a prescribed drug regimen. Similarly, both the therapeutic and side-effects of a drug can affect nutrient intake, metabolism and requirements and, ultimately, nutritional status (Table 3 below).

Food (or individual nutrients) can have a marked effect on drug effectiveness by increasing, decreasing or simply delaying absorption. Food can also influence the rate of drug metabolism by either increasing or decreasing the production of the drug-metabolising enzymes or by influencing splanchnic-hepatic blood flow. Therapeutic efficacy is affected when, for example, a food delays or prevents drug absorption or accelerates the rate of drug metabolism or excretion, while a toxic reaction is possible when a food increases the absorption of a drug or inhibits its metabolism or excretion. It is, therefore, important to be aware of the possible interactions between drugs and nutrients and the potential effects on both patient nutrition and on drug therapy itself.

Relationships between nutrition and drug therapy

The many problems that may be associated with drug therapy can affect any patient. There are, however, some situations in which the effects of drugs may be particularly significant in nutritional terms. For example, the side-effects associated with cancer chemotherapy may significantly affect food consumption and nutritional sta-

Table 3. Effects of drug action on nutritional status

Alterations in food consumption	
	Appetite changes
	Alterations in the perception of taste/smell
	Decreased secretion of saliva
	Gastric irritation or discomfort
	Nausea and vomiting
Alterations in the absorption of nutrients	
Luminal effects	Altered gastrointestinal pH
	Changed gastrointestinal motility
	Altered activity of the bile acids
	Binding of nutrients, thus preventing absorption
Mucosal effects	Inactivation of enzyme systems
	Reduction in the absorptive due to damage to gastrointestinal mucosal cells' surface area
	Alterations in the metabolism and/or utilisation of nutrients
	Alteration in the pattern of nutrient excretion

Notes

Table 4. Examples of drug effects on nutrient absorption

Primary effects	Drug	Effect
Effects within the lumen		
Absorption	Cholestyramine	Lowered folic acid
Precipitation	Aluminium hydroxide	Lowered phosphate
Binding	Tetracycline	Lowered calcium
Change in pH	Sodium bicarbonate	Lowered folic acid
Enzyme inhibition	Sulphasalazine	Lowered folic acid
Solubilisation	Mineral oils	Lowered fat-soluble vitamins
Change in motility		
Decreased gastric emptying	Anticholinergic agents	Increased riboflavin
Decreased intestinal transit	Cathartic agents	General malabsorption
	Bisacodyl	Lowered glucose
Mucosal damage		
Cytotoxicity	Neomycin	Lowered fat
	Colchicine	
	Methotrexate	Lowered calcium
Secondary effects		
Maldigestion	Alcohol	Lowered fat through impaired bile acid secretion
Non-gastrointestinal enzyme inhibition	Isoniazid	Lowered calcium through inhibition of vitamin D metabolism
Drug-induced vitamin deficiency	Alcohol	Lowered thiamine due to malabsorption of folate

tus (Holmes, 1997), while radiotherapy may also interfere with the ability to eat and drink (Holmes, 1996).

Chronic drug use may potentiate nutrient deficiencies due to decreased nutrient intake, malabsorption, hyper-excretion of nutrients, increased nutrient catabolism or impaired nutrient utilisation.

Some drugs may, themselves, directly influence nutritional status, while the intake of some nutrients may contribute to the response to individual drugs (see, for example, Roe, 1985; Rikans, 1986). For example, some drugs can cause anorexia and thereby reduce food and, hence, nutrient intake.

Drugs may also influence the absorption, metabolism and elimination of nutrients due to direct actions on either the gastrointestinal tract (primary effects) and/or on other organs, such as the liver (secondary effects) (Table 4 above).

Drugs may affect nutrient metabolism in two ways: they may increase nutrient catabolism or, alternatively, may inhibit enzymes essential to drug metabolism and/or utilisation. For example, the antitubercular drug isoniazid and the cardiovascular drug hydralazine may cause deficiency of pyridoxine (vitamin B_6) by inhibiting the action of the enzyme pyridoxal kinase while sulphasalazine may decrease serum folic acid. Other drugs (for example, phenytoin, phenobarbitone and carbamazepine) cause an increase in the activity of hepatic enzymes, resulting in an increased breakdown of nutrients such as folate (folic acid).

Nutrient deficiencies (for example, protein, folic acid, vitamin C and potassium) may compound such effects so that the products of drug metabolism and, in some cases, unchanged drugs, are excreted in both the bile and the urine (Dickerson, 1988). Similarly, any condition that results in a decline in renal function may mean that drugs and their degradation products are retained in the body for prolonged periods (Blackford, 1995), thus prolonging both their therapeutic and deleterious effects.

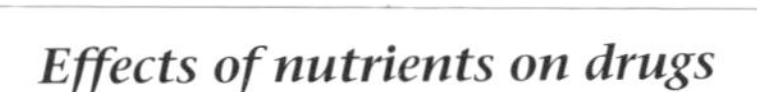

Notes

Effects of nutrients on drugs

It is quite clear that drug absorption may be influenced by food.

In general, drugs taken with food are absorbed more slowly; at times, total absorption may be reduced, primarily because of delayed gastric emptying and consequent dilution. Such reductions in drug absorption may mean that effective drug levels cannot be reached and the therapeutic effect is reduced.

Alternatively, slow absorption may act as a form of 'sustained release', thus prolonging drug effects. Therefore nutrients may substantially interfere with pharmacotherapeutic goals, affecting the bioavailability and distribution of a number of orally administered drugs (Kirk, 1995). The resultant clinical effects may, therefore, range from insignificance to an adverse drug reaction or to a failure of therapy (Blackford, 1995).

Gastric emptying is also delayed by hot meals, by solutions of high viscosity and, to a lesser extent, by high protein and carbohydrate foods (Dickerson, 1988). Prolonged retention of drugs in the acid environment of the stomach will tend to accelerate the dissolution of basic compounds while delaying that of acidic drugs. Thus the timing of drug administration in relation to food may have both clinical and economic implications. This must be considered seriously when planning any therapeutic regime.

In general, drugs should not be taken with meals unless they cause significant gastrointestinal distress, when the presence of food can decrease distress/discomfort. Because gastrointestinal distress or discomfort is a common consequence of many drugs (for example, non-steroidal anti-inflammatory agents and steroids) 'trade-offs' must sometimes be made and such drugs must be given with food even if absorption is decreased. This may, in itself, help to improve food consumption.

When a rapid effect is required, drugs are given on an empty stomach (for example, analgesics, hypnotics and anti-infective agents). Studies show altered absorption responses in 77–93% of drugs when food is present in the digestive tract (Murray and Healy, 1991). In other cases, the absorption, safety and effectiveness of drugs may be enhanced by fluid intake, especially water (for example, aspirin, iron preparations, penicillamine and many antibiotics).

As a general principle, the recommended timing for drug therapy is one hour before or two hours after meals unless the medication causes gastrointestinal disturbances when taken on an empty stomach. This enhances drug absorption and decreases interference with nutrient absorption.

Surgery

Surgery is often associated with prolonged fasting both pre- and postoperatively. Preoperative diagnostic procedures and blood tests frequently require patients to fast or receive clear fluids only, thus militating against optimal nutrient intake (Garrow, 1994). This may be exacerbated by unnecessarily prolonged preoperative starvation.

It has been shown that many patients are regularly starved for significantly longer than is physiologically necessary (Maclean and Renwick, 1993; Greenfield et al, 1997) even though this has been shown to be both illogical and unnecessary since the fasting stomach will, in any case, secrete up to 50ml of gastric juice per hour (Guyton, 1986), while clear fluids rapidly leave the stomach of healthy people; about half the volume disappears within 10–20 minutes (Sutherland et al, 1987). Thus, although patients who are likely to have delayed gastric emptying (through underlying disease or drug therapy) should not drink before anaesthesia or intravenous sedation, there is now overwhelming evidence to suggest that other patients should be allowed to drink clear fluids up to two hours before this is given (Greenfield et al, 1997).

This, combined with at least some degree of postoperative catabolism, can be particularly important in patients who are already malnourished or whose nutritional status is marginal and may influence the outcome of surgical procedures.

Notes

Indeed, a number of studies have clearly demonstrated the effect of undernutrition in this situation. For example, Windsor and Hill (1988) showed that, in those undergoing significant gastrointestinal resection, malnourished patients developed four times as many complications (primarily pneumonia), were twice as likely to develop some form of sepsis and were generally likely to remain in hospital for longer periods.

Preoperative nutritional support should be considered whenever elective surgery is contemplated, as this is known to reduce morbidity, especially in older patients (Hirsch, 1995). This is particularly true when preoperative starvation is likely to extend beyond three to five days and major surgery is likely to involve the gastrointestinal tract, pancreas and/or biliary tract (Buzby, 1988). However, if sepsis is present nutritional support is unlikely to improve either the clinical or nutritional outcome, but it has been shown that the duration of support can influence postoperative outcome. This has been described as follows:

- Three days of support may shorten hospital stay (Rumley et al, 1987; Young et al, 1989);
- In patients with a positive nitrogen balance, plasma transferrin and prealbumin return to normal levels within one to two weeks, provided no infection is present (Church and Hill, 1987);
- Wound-healing may be returned to normal (Haydock and Hill, 1987);
- Immunocompetence may be restored after two to five weeks in severely malnourished people (Bistrian et al, 1976).

Since nutritional support in the postoperative period should be planned on an individual basis and related to the type of surgery performed, the nutritional care of patients following surgery will vary. Certain general principles can, however, be applied.

Following surgery a combination of starvation and increased catabolism, stimulated by the sympathetic nervous system, together with the release of glucocorticoid hormones, will cause loss of body protein and fat (Table 5 below); The extent of such losses depends on the following:

- The preoperative nutritional status;
- The extent of surgery;
- The presence/absence of postoperative complications, particularly sepsis (Hill, 1988).

Hill et al (1978) report that the average tissue loss following rectal surgery is 4kg, of which 1.3kg is fat, 1kg is protein (lean body mass) and 1.8kg is water. Others report similar findings after any major surgery. Such losses may be masked, at least to some degree, by retention of sodium and water, with the effect that weight loss may not become apparent until diuresis occurs — three to seven days after surgery. Such losses may be exacerbated by postoperative starvation.

Table 5. The metabolic response to stress or injury

Stimulation of the sympathetic nervous system results in release of adrenaline and noradrenaline which: increase heart rate and cardiac output, oxygen consumption and metabolic rate; enhance the breakdown of glucose; redistribute blood flow to ensure that essential organs are perfused; reduce uptake of glucose by tissues and gastric motility and digestion; cause pupils to dilate; cause constriction of sphincters in gastro-intestinal tract and bladder; arouse the central nervous system	Stimulation of the anterior pituitary gland and adrenal cortex result in the release of cortisol and other glucorticoids which: stimulate production of 'new' glucose (gluconeo-genesis) and mobilisation of fat and protein; reduce tissue utilisation of glucose; suppress the inflammatory response; inhibit granulation tissue; enhance expansion of extracellular fluid volume through retention of sodium and water

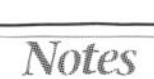

Table 6. Classification of catabolism (after Rutten et al, 1975)

Clinical state	Degree of catabolism	Urea nitrogen (g/day)	Increase of metabolic rate over BMR (%)	Total energy requirement (kcal)
Bedrest	1° (normal)	less than 3	none	1,800
Uncomplicated surgery	2° (mild)	5–10	0–20	1,800–2,000
Multiple fractures or trauma	3° (moderate)	10–15	20–50	2,200–2,700
Acute major infection or burns	3° (severe)	more than 15	30–125	2,700–4,000 (or more)

Drainage or fistulae, vomiting or diarrhoea may exacerbate this still further and so exhaust body protein and fat stores.

Energy needs, therefore, are increased after surgery. Following uncomplicated elective surgery the increase will be in the region of 10% but, if the surgery was preceded by trauma or multiple fractures, the increase may be anywhere between 10–25% (Table 6 above) (Rutten et al, 1975).

If insufficient nutrients — particularly carbohydrate or fat — are available, body protein will be broken down to provide energy. Exudates and discharges will exacerbate protein loss. The net effect of these events may have serious consequences, causing oedema, inhibiting wound-healing, impairing immunocompetence and preventing resumption of gastrointestinal activity. Protein loss also impedes regeneration of haemoglobin and delays convalescence by preventing restoration of muscular strength.

Postoperative patients were, in the past, supported primarily by means of intravenous infusions designed more to restore fluid and electrolyte balance than to maintain nutritional status. Enteral feeding was not permitted until bowel sounds were heard, as the risk of postoperative ileus was considered a contraindication to feeding. It is now known that enteral feeding can be safely administered into the jejunum during this period and Yeung et al (1979) found that an additional 2000kcal/day provided through this route did not impair voluntary food consumption.

Although Taylor and Goodinson-McLaren (1993) suggested that it was probably unnecessary to give either pre- or postoperative nutritional support to previously well-nourished patients undergoing uncomplicated or minor surgery, it is clear that malnourished patients, or those about to undergo major surgery necessitating prolonged fasting, should be considered for nutritional support.

Vitamin and/or mineral supplementation is not, however, usually needed by previously healthy individuals undergoing minor surgery, but older adults may benefit from such support (Hirsch, 1995).

Patients fasting for longer than a total of four days during the perioperative period and those having major surgery, especially if poorly prepared for it, usually require therapeutic doses of vitamins.

Psychosocial influences on food consumption

Eating is often a symbolic experience embedded in lifelong patterns and cultural preferences (Holzapfel et al, 1996), so that the environment during meal times can be of extreme importance. This extends beyond the physical into social and psychological arenas and incorporates the type of food offered to individuals.

Even in health, food intake is heavily influenced by a wide variety of social, cultural and psychological factors (Novin and van der Weele, 1977; Holmes, 1986). These may become increasingly important in illness. Awareness of the factors involved, and understanding of the role of food

Notes

habits and their contribution to eating patterns and behaviour, is central to helping patients to eat appropriately or to comply with the demands of a dietary prescription. Food habits and eating behaviour in turn determine food choice and, therefore, nutrient intake.

Food habits represent the adoption of social, cultural and religious values of the society in which we live. Their development starts in infancy, continuing throughout childhood into adult life. During childhood, dependency on others for food provision significantly influences the foods available. Children tend to develop a taste for the foods their mother likes or provides for them. During continuing growth and development such behaviour is reinforced, creating the basis of food choices and setting the pattern for future eating habits. A gradually increasing exposure to a wide range of additional influences may modify these habits, as foods provided are seen as examples of what is both appropriate and nutritionally acceptable.

Similarly, cultural and traditional standards influence eating behaviour. Their influence is indirect during early life but becomes increasingly marked as a child gets older. All societies possess a unique culture with its own traditions and customs which, in turn, determine appropriate behaviours. Therefore, although societal influences are subconscious, culture becomes a way of life. Few people are aware of the extent to which such factors influence their life.

In terms of food, all cultures identify those foods that are acceptable; many also dictate the manner in which foods can or should be prepared — for example, kosher food or halal meat.

Religion may be a particularly important cultural determinant of food acceptability and be associated with particular eating practices or food consumption. Since consumption of specific foods, or foods prepared in a particular way, may demonstrate religious faith, this may be of immense importance to individual patients.

Similarly, for those from other cultures adherence to familiar food habits may be important in creating feelings of security and stability. Failure to adhere to religious practices can, therefore, cause considerable distress and resentment; security is threatened and food refusal more likely (Farb and Armelagos, 1980). Illness does not provide the opportunity to attempt to change long-established food habits.

Food habits can also contribute to the meeting of safety needs, such as those for protection and predictability. These may be met by expressing a preference for familiar foods and avoiding those that are unfamiliar and/or disliked. Thus, in an unfamiliar environment, such as a hospital ward, the presentation of familiar and acceptable foods can do a great deal to reassure a patient; it is also likely to encourage food consumption.

Indeed, Steptoe et al (1995) showed that familiarity was one of the most important factors underlying food selection. The others were general health, mood, convenience, sensory appeal, natural content, price, weight control and ethical concerns.

Food has many emotional meanings over and above those of meeting nutritional needs. Such meanings are often deeply embedded in individual ideology, as a result of which food habits are often highly resistant to change. It also shows that the apparently simple act of satisfying hunger and meeting nutritional needs is, in fact, a highly complex activity. This may create significant difficulties for hospitalised patients. Therefore, although NHS Executive catering guidelines (NHS Executive, 1996) suggest that the foods offered should meet the preferences and dietary needs of all patients, this can be difficult to achieve. Considerable ingenuity and flexibility may be required to provide an appropriate and nutritionally adequate diet for individual patients.

Effects and consequences of malnutrition

Although malnutrition significantly influences the recovery of health, clinical surveys continue to reveal an

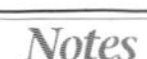

unacceptably high incidence in hospitals (for example, Larsson et al, 1990; Moy et al, 1990; McWhirter and Pennington, 1994). Yet the clinical consequences of malnutrition have long been recognised and lead to increased complication rates and prolonged in-patient treatment, as a result of which the costs of hospital care are significantly increased (Pettigrew and Hill, 1986; Robinson et al, 1987; Larsson et al, 1990). Readmission rates are also increased (Williams and Fitton, 1988; Sullivan, 1992; Tierney et al, 1994).

Obvious effects of malnutrition include weight loss, depletion of subcutaneous fat, progressive muscle-wasting, apathy, malaise and lethargy (Brozek, 1990). Such symptoms exacerbate the condition, promoting a further loss of appetite. A vicious circle of uninterest in food and apathy may develop from which it can be difficult to escape.

The decline in body mass, combined with physical weakness, inhibits mobility and increases the liability to venous stasis, deep-vein thrombosis and the development of pressure sores (Holmes et al, 1987). Respiration may be impaired as respiratory muscles weaken (Arora and Rochester, 1962; Doekel et al, 1976), making it difficult for patients to cough or expectorate effectively and increasing the susceptibility to chest infection. It also reduces cardiac function, with a consequent likelihood of cardiac failure (Heymsfield et al, 1978). Immunocompetence declines, resulting in increased susceptibility to infection (Chandra, 1990) that, in turn, further reduces nutritional status (Bistrian et al, 1977). Small intestinal changes (Stanfield et al, 1965) lead to malabsorption, possibly exacerbated by an associated reduction in pancreatic secretion.

Wound-healing is prevented and dehiscence is common (Windsor and Hill, 1988). The tolerance to stressful therapies, such as cancer chemotherapy and radiotherapy (Goodinson, 1987; Holmes, 1996; 1997) is reduced, and severely malnourished patients requiring surgery are at an increased risk of postoperative complications (Windsor and Hill, 1988). Acute medical patients are no less at risk and episodes of sepsis more commonly affect the undernourished patient (Potter et al, 1995).

As a result of these deleterious effects malnourished patients often have lower morale and a reduced will to recover. They may find it difficult to participate in self-care activities or to benefit from advice designed to promote or maintain future health (Silk, 1994). These effects may, in turn, significantly decrease both the desire and the ability to eat, reducing nutritional status still further and again increasing the cost of health care. Indeed, the cost of treating a malnourished patient experiencing a major complication is four times that of a normal uncomplicated recovery (Reilly et al, 1987) and, in general medical wards, results in a doubling of hospital charges.

Summary

Malnutrition clearly affects significant numbers of hospital patients in whom it delays recovery and increases the cost of hospitalisation; it also increases the risk of mortality. Its prevention must, therefore, be a primary aim in health care and clearly requires collaboration between all health care professionals. The difficulty is that no one group of health care professionals can or should accept responsibility for the nutrition of the general hospital patient — it is truly a multidisciplinary aspect of care.

Although nurses cannot accept sole responsibility for this aspect of care they can and should play a central role in patient feeding and in identifying vulnerable patients. Recognition of the risk of malnutrition must, for the majority of patients, rest with nurses. It is, therefore, incumbent on nurses to ensure that their knowledge of nutrition enables them to fulfil this role. **NT**

Notes

References

Allison, S. (1996) The management of malnutrition in hospital. *Proceedings of the Nutrition Society*; 55: 3, 855–862.

American Society of Parenteral and Enteral Nutrition (1993) Guidelines for the use of enteral and parenteral nutrition in adult and pediatric patients. *Journal of Enteral and Parenteral Nutrition*; 17 (Suppl 4): 1SA–52SA.

Anderson, M.A., Collins, G., Davis, G., Bivins, B. A. (1985) Malnutrition and length of stay — a relationship? *Henry Ford Hospital Medical Journal*; 33: 4, 190–193.

Arora, N.S., Rochester, D.F. (1982) Respiratory muscle strength and maximal voluntary ventilation in undernourished patients. *American Review of Respiratory Diseases*; 126; 1: 5–8.

Association of Community Health Councils (1997) *Hungry in Hospital?* London: Association of Community Health Councils for England and Wales.

Bastow, M.D., Rawlings, J., Allison, S.P. (1983) Benefits of supplementary tube-feeding after fractured neck of femur: a randomised controlled trial. *British Medical Journal*; 287: 6405, 1589–1592.

Bistrian, B.R., Sherman, M., Blackburn , G.L. (1977) Cellular immunity in adult marasmus. *Archives in Medicine*; 137: 10, 1408–1411.

Bistrian, B.R., Blackburn, G.L., Hallowell, E., Heddle, R. (1974) Protein status of general surgical patients. *Journal of the American Medical Association*; 230: 6, 858–860.

Bistrian, B.R., Blackburn, G.L., Vitale, J., et al (1976) Prevalence of malnutrition in general medical patients. *Journal of the American Medical Association* 235: 15, 1567–1570.

Blackford, M.S. (1995) Drug therapy in older adults: effects of altered pharmacokinetics and pharmacodynamics. *Ohio Nurses Review;* 70: 2, 13–17.

British Dietetic Association (1996) *Malnutrition in Hospital. Position Paper.* Birmingham: British Dietetic Association.

Brozek, J. (1990). Effects of generalised malnutrition on personality. *Nutrition*; 6: 389–395.

Butterworth, C.E. (1974) The skeleton in the hospital closet. *Nutrition Today*; 8: 4–8.

Buzby, G.P. (1988) Preoperative nutritional support. In: Jeejeebhoy, K.N. (ed) *Current Therapy in Nutrition*. Oxford: Blackwell/Decker.

Carr, E.K., Mitchell, J.R. (1991) A comparison of the mealtime care given to patients by nurses using two different meal delivery systems. *International Journal of Nursing Studies*; 28: 1, 19–25.

Chandra, R. K. (1990) The relation between immunology, nutrition and disease in elderly people. *Age and Ageing;* 19: 4 (Suppl 1), S25–31.

Church, J.M., Hill, G.L. (1987) Assessing the efficacy of intravenous nutrition in surgical patients — dynamic nutritional assessment using plasma proteins. *Journal of Parenteral and Enteral Nutrition*; 11: 135–139.

Clark, J. (1980) Introduction (nutrition and health). *Nursing*; 11: 463–464.

Closs, S.J. (1993) Malnutrition: the key to pressure sores? *Nursing Standard*; 89: 20, 58–60.

Department of Health (1992) *The Health of Elderly People: An Epidemiological Overview (Central Health Monitoring Unit Epidemiological Overview Series, Volume 1).* London: HMSO.

Department of Health (1994) *Nutrition: Core Curriculum for Nutrition in the Education of Health Professionals*. London: Department of Health.

Deutekom, E.J., Philipsen, H., Ten Hoor, F., Abu-Saad, H. (1991) Plate-waste-producing situations on nursing wards. *International Journal of Nursing Studies*; 28: 2, 163–174.

Dickerson, J.W. (1988) The interrelationships of nutrition and drugs. In: Dickerson, J.W., Lee, H.A. (eds) *Nutrition in the Clinical Management of Disease*. London: Edward Arnold.

Dickerson, J. W., Fekkes, J., Goodinson, S.M. (1986) Postoperative food intake in elderly fracture patients. *Proceedings of the Nutrition Society*; 45: 7A.

Dickerson, J.W. (1986) Hospital-induced malnutrition. In: Holmes, S. (ed), *Nutrition in Nursing Practice. Conference Proceedings*. Guildford, Surrey: University of Surrey, Division of Nursing Studies.

Doekel, R.C., Zwillich, C.W., Scoggin, C. et al (1976) Clinical semi-starvation: depression of hypoxic ventilatory response. *New England Journal of Medicine*; 295: 7, 358–361.

Eastwood, M. (1997) Hospital food. *New England Journal of Medicine*; 336: 17, 1261.

ENB (1995) *Nutrition for Life: Issues for Debate in the Development of Education Programmes*. London: ENB.

Farb, P., Armelagos, G. (1980) *Consuming Passions: The Anthropology of Eating*. Boston, Mass: Houghton-Mifflin.

Garrow, J. (1994) Starvation in hospital (Letter to the editor). *British Medical Journal*; 308: 6934, 934.

Goodinson, S.M. (1987) Assessment of nutritional status. *Professional Nurse*; 2: 11, 367–369.

Greenfield, S.M., Webster G.J., Vicary, F.R. (1997) Drinking before sedation: preoperative fasting should be the exception rather than the rule. *British Medical Journal*; 314: 7075, 162.

Guyton, A.C. (1986) *Textbook of Medical Physiology.* Philadelphia, Pa: W.B. Saunders.

Haydock, D.A., Hill, G.L. (1987) Impaired wound-healing in surgical patients with varying degrees of malnutrition. *Journal of Parenteral and Enteral Nutrition*; 10: 550–554.

Heymsfield, S.B., Bethel, R.A., Asley, J.D. (1978) Cardiac abnormalities in cachectic patients before and during nutritional repletion. *American Heart Journal*; 95: 5, 584–594.

Hill, G.L., Blackett, R.I., Pickford, I., et al (1977) Malnutrition in surgical patients - an unrecognised problem. *Lancet*; 1: 8013, 689–692.

Hill, G.L. (1988) The perioperative patient. In: Kinney J.M., Jeejeebhoy, K.N., Hill, G. L., Owens, C.E. (eds) *Nutrition and Metabolism in Patient Care.* Philadelphia, Pa: W.B. Saunders.

Hill, G.L., McCarthy, T.D., Collins, J.P., Smith, A.H. (1978) A new method for the rapid measurement of body composition in critically ill surgical patients. *British Journal of Surgery*; 65: 10, 732–735.

Hirsch, C.H. (1995) When your patient needs surgery: how planning can avoid complications. *Geriatrics*; 50: 2, 39–44.

Holmes, R., MacChiano, K., Shangiani, S. et al (1987) Combating pressures — nutritionally. *American Journal of Nursing;* 87: 1301–1303.

Holmes, S. (1996) *Radiotherapy: A Guide for Practice.* Leatherhead, Surrey: Asset Books.

Holmes, S. (1997) *Cancer Chemotherapy: A Guide for Practice.* Leatherhead, Surrey: Asset Books.

Holmes, S. (1986) Determinants of food intake. *Nursing*; 3: 7, 260–264.

Holmes, S., Dickerson, J.W. (1987) Malignant disease: nutritional implications of disease and treatment. *Cancer and Metastasis Reviews*; 6: 3, 357–381.

Holmes, S. (1994) Nutrition and older people: a matter of concern. *Nursing Times*; 90: 42, 31–33.

Holzapfel, S.K., Ramirez, R.F., Layton, M.S. et al (1996) Feeder position and food and fluid consumed by nursing home residents. *Journal of Gerontological Nursing;* 22: 4, 6–12.

Keller, H.H. (1993) Malnutrition in institutionalised elderly: how and why? *Journal of the American Geriatrics Society*; 41: 11, 1212–1218.

Kirk, S.F. (1995) Adequacy of meals served and consumed at a long-stay hospital for the elderly. *Care of the Elderly*; 2: 2, 77–80.

Larsson, J., Unosson, M., Ek, A-C. (1990) Effect of dietary supplementation on nutritional status and clinical outcome on 501 geriatric patients — a randomised study. *Clinical Nutrition*; 9: 179–184.

Lennard-Jones, J.E. (1992) *A Positive Approach to Nutrition as Treatment: Report of a Working Party on the Role of Enteral and Parenteral Feeding in Hospital and at Home.* London: Kings' Fund.

Maclean, A.R., Renwick, C. (1993) Audit of preoperative starvation. *Anaesthesia*; 48: 2, 164–166.

Maras, M.L. , Adolphi, C.L. (1985) Ethnic tailoring improves dietary compliance. *Diabetes Education*; 11: 4, 47–50.

McCamish, M. (1993) Malnutrition and nutrition support interventions: costs, benefits and outcomes (editorial). *Nutrition*; 9: 556-557.

McWhirter, J.P, Pennington, C.R. (1994) Incidence and recognition of malnutrition in hospitals. *British Medical Journal*; 308: 6934, 945–948.

Mennell, S., Murcott, A., Otterloo, A.H. (1994) *The Sociology of Food, Eating, Diet and Culture.* London: Sage Publications.

Moy, R.J., Smallman, S., Booth, I.W. (1990) Malnutrition in a UK children's hospital. *Journal of Human Nutrition and Dietetics*; 3: 93–70.

Mulliner, C.M., Spiby, H., Fraser, R.B. (1995) A study exploring midwives' education in, knowledge of and attitudes to nutrition in pregnancy. *Midwifery*; 11: 1, 7–41.

Murray, J.J., Healy, D.M. (1991) Drug-mineral interactions: a new responsibility for the hospital dietitian. *Journal of the American Dietetic Association*; 91: 1, 66–70.

NHS Executive (1996) *Guidelines for Hospital Catering.* Leeds: NHSE.

Novin, D., van der Weele, D.A. (1977) Visceral involvement in feeding. *Progress in Physiology and Psychology*; 7: 193–241.

Older, M.W., Dickerson, J.W. (1982) Thiamine and the elderly orthopaedic patient. *Age and Ageing*; 11: 2, 107.

Parker, D., Emmett, P.M., Heaton, K.W. (1992) Final-year medical students' knowledge of practical nutrition. *Journal of the Royal Society of Medicine*; 85: 6, 338.

Patients' Association (1993) *Catering for Patients in Hospital. Environmental Issues*

Notes

Notes

Working Group. London: Patients' Association.

Pettigrew, R.A., Hill, G.L. (1986) Indicators of surgical risk and clinical judgement. *British Journal of Surgery*; 73: 1, 47–51.

Philen, R.M., Ortiz,, D.I., Auerbach, S.B., Falk, H. (1992) Survey of advertising for nutritional supplements in health and body building magazines. *Journal of the American Medical Association*; 268: 8, 1008–1011.

Potter, J., Klipstein, K., Reilly, J.J., Roberts, M. (1995) The nutritional status and clinical course of acute admissions to a geriatric unit. *Age and Ageing*; 24: 2, 131–136.

Puxty, J.H. (1985) Infections, vitamins and confusion in the elderly. In: Kemm, J.R., Ancill, R.J. (eds) *Vitamin Deficiency in the Elderly*. Oxford: Blackwell Scientific.

Rademaker, J.W. , Richards, C., Marsham, J., et al (1996) Management of malnutrition in the elderly: a clinical audit. *Proceedings of the Nutrition Society*; 56: 2, 175A.

Rana, S.K., Bray, J., Menzies, G.W., et al. (1992) Short-term benefits of post-operative oral dietary supplements in surgical patients. *Clinical Nutrition*; 11: 337–344.

Reilly, H.M. 1996) Screening for nutritional risk. *Proceedings of the Nutrition Society*; 55: 3, 841–843.

Reilly, J.J., Hull, S.F., Albert, N. (1987) Economic impact of malnutrition: a model system for hospitalised patients. *Journal of Parenteral and Enteral Nutrition*; 12: 372–376.

Rikans, L.E. (1986) Drugs and nutrition in old age. *Life Science*; 39: 12, 1027–1036.

Robinson, G., Goldstein, M., Levine, G.M. (1987) Impact of nutritional status on DRG length of stay. *Journal of Parenteral and Enteral Nutrition*; 11: 45–51.

Roe, D.A. (1985) Drug effects on nutrient absorption, transport and metabolism. *Drug-Nutrient Interactions*; 4: 1–2, 117–135.

Rumley, I.D., Lineaweaver, W.C., Davis, J.M. (1987) Low residue nutritional supplementation as an adjunct to mechanical preparation for surgical treatment of the colon. *Surgery, Gynaecology and Obstetrics*; 164: 4, 345–350.

Rutten, P., Blackburn, G.L., Flatt J.P. et al (1975) Determination of optimal hyperalimentation infusion rate. *Journal of Surgical Research*; 18: 5, 477–479.

Schorah, C.J., Newill, A., Scott, D.L., Morgan, D.B. (1979) Clinical effects of vitamin C in elderly patients with low blood vitamin C levels. *Lancet*; 1: 8113, 403–405.

Scott, A., Skerratt, S., Adam, A. (1998) *Nutrition for the Critically Ill: A Practical Handbook*. London: Arnold.

Silk, D.B. (ed) (1994) *Organisation of Nutritional Support in Hospitals. A Report by a Working Party of the British Association for Parenteral and Enteral Nutrition*. Maidenhead, Berks: BAPEN.

Simon, S. (1991) A survey of the nutritional adequacy of meals served and eaten by patients. *Nursing Practice*; 4: 2, 7–11.

Sonies, B.C., Parent, L.J., Morrish, K., Baum, B.J. (1988) Durational aspects of the oral-pharyngeal phase of swallow in normal adults. *Dysphagia*; 3: 1, 1–10.

Steptoe, A., Pollard, J.M., Wardle, J. (1995) Development of a measure of the motives underlying the selection of food: the food choice questionnaire. *Appetite*; 25: 3, 267–284.

Stiles, J. (1998) Relative nourishment. *Nursing Standard*; 12: 50, 25.

Sullivan, D. H. (1992) Risk factors for early hospital readmission in a select population of geriatric rehabilitation patients: the significance of nutritional status. *Journal of the American Geriatrics Society*; 40: 8, 792–798.

Sutherland, A.D., Malthy, J.R., Sale, J.P., Reid, C.R. (1987) The effect of preoperative oral fluid and ranitidine on gastric fluid volume and pH. *Canadian Journal of Anaestheology*; 34: 2, 117–121.

Taylor, S., Goodinson-McLaren, S. (1993) *Nutrition Support: A Team Approach*. London: Wolfe Publishing.

Tierney, A.J., Worth, A., Closs, S.J. et al (1994) Older patients' experiences of discharge from hospital. *Nursing Times*; 90: 21, 36–39.

Tucker, H. (1996) Cost containment through nutritional intervention. *Nutrition Reviews*; 54: 4, Pt1, 111–112.

Wainwright, H. (1978) Feeding problems in elderly disabled patients. *Nursing Times*; 74: 13, 542–543.

Williams, E.I., Fitton, F. (1988) Factors affecting early unplanned readmission of elderly patients to hospital. *British Medical Journal*; 297: 6651, 784–787.

Williams, C.M., Driver, L.T., Older, J., Dickerson, J.W. (1989) A controlled trial of sip-feed supplements in elderly orthopaedic patients. *European Journal of Clinical Nutrition*; 43: 4, 267–274.

Wilson, D.O. (1990) Metabolic rate and weight loss in chronic obstructive lung disease. *Journal of Parenteral and Enteral Nutrition*; 14: 7–11.

Windsor, J.A., Hill, G.L. (1988) Protein depletion and surgical risk. *Australian and*

New Zealand Journal of Surgery; 58: 9, 711–715.

Yeung, C.K., Young, G.A., Hackett, A.F., Hill, G.L. (1979) Fine-needle catheter jejunostomy — an assessment of a new method of nutritional support after major gastrointestinal surgery. *British Journal of Surgery*; 66: 10, 727–732.

Young, G.A., Zeiderman, M.R. , Thompson, M., McMahon, M.J. (1989) Influence of postoperative intravenous nutrition upon hepatic protein synthesis and plasma and amino acids. *Journal of Parenteral and Enteral Nutrition*; 13: 727–732.

Notes

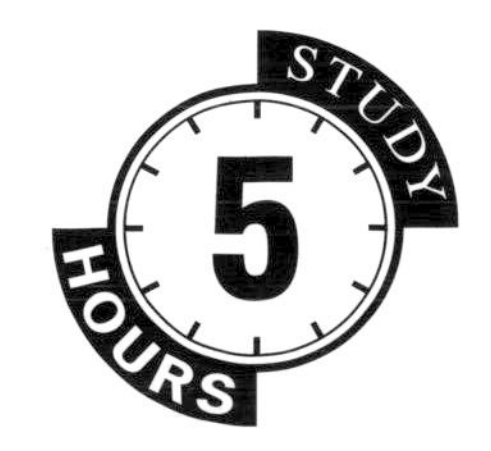

Notes